MiNDFULNESS FOR KiDS
iN 10 MiNUTES A DAY

MINDFULNESS FOR KIDS

in 10 Minutes a Day

Simple Exercises to Feel
CALM, FOCUSED, AND HAPPY

MAURA BRADLEY

Illustrated by Cait Brennan

ROCKRIDGE
PRESS

For my kids,
EMMA, **WILL**, and **MAEVE**,
who taught me the true meaning
of learning to live in the present
moment and to see the joy in the little
things. And to my husband, Derek, my
biggest supporter and my best friend.
I love you all more than you
will ever know.

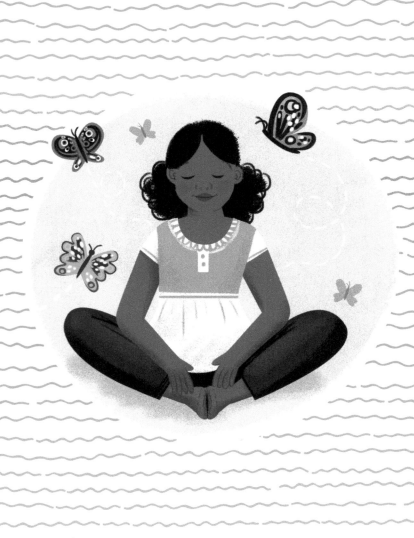

CONTENTS

WHAT IS MINDFULNESS, ANYWAY?

Mindfulness Is Your Friend

Mindfulness is something you may or may not have heard of before. People use the word *mindful* to describe many things. But what is mindfulness, anyway? It means paying attention to where you are, what you're doing, and how you're feeling—all at the same time. But how do we do that? And, more important, why?

We can practice mindfulness in many different ways. For example, we can use one of our five senses. Let's begin with sight. Stop what you're doing right now and look around. Notice what you can see and notice your surroundings. This is mindfulness. You just practiced being aware of where you are in the moment. Simple, right?

Take it a step further. Now that you have noticed where you are, notice how you are feeling. Not just your emotions, like happy, mad, or sad, but also how you feel physically. Are you warm? Cold? Can you feel your feet on the ground? Taking a moment to notice how you feel in your body is also mindfulness.

Now for the really cool part. By stopping to notice where we are and how we are feeling, we are bringing our attention to the present moment. When you are present, your mind will not think about worries from the past, like something you regret doing or saying. Your mind will not think about future worries either, like an upcoming test or sports game.

Practicing mindfulness can improve all areas of your life by reducing anxiety and worry. It can help you do better in school, handle stress, have better relationships with friends and family, get better sleep, and provide overall happiness! In this book, you will learn how to train your brain so that you can begin practicing mindfulness in just 10 minutes a day.

Making Mindfulness Stick

Mindfulness can be simple and challenging at the same time. But the more time you take to practice being mindful, the easier it will become. What do you do if you want to get better at something, whether it's baseball, singing, or math? You practice! It works the same way with mindfulness. It doesn't have to take a lot of time out of your day. Practicing for 10 minutes in the morning, afternoon, or evening will help you develop a habit. The benefits of this simple practice will last a lifetime.

Research has shown that it takes somewhere between 21 and 60 days to form a new habit. This book has you covered with 60 mindfulness exercises for you to try. By picking just one short exercise per day, you will be well on your way to forming a habit of mindfulness. Want to do better in class? Focus on schoolwork? Learn how to calm your fear or anxiety all by yourself? You can do this and so much more with regular mindfulness practice. Give it a try!

How It All Works

This book is divided into three sections: Morning, Midday, and Night. You will find different ways to practice mindfulness at any point in the day. Maybe your mornings are a blur of alarm clocks ringing, a quick breakfast, and rushing out the door for school. If that is the case, you may not think it's the best time for you to practice mindfulness. But guess what? You might be surprised to learn that you can be mindful during those super-busy mornings! Taking a short mindful break from your usual chaotic routine may be the perfect way to start your day. Scheduling your mindfulness practice each day will help you fit it in, no matter how busy you may be. This book is designed to give you options. Every day, you can pick any time to practice that works for you!

WHERE DO I START?

Each section of the book contains 20 mindfulness practices. There are four types of exercises:

 Calm exercises help you relax.

 Focus exercises help you pay attention.

 Reconnect exercises help you notice your feelings or emotions.

 Respond exercises help you react to negative emotions or events in a mindful way.

You can choose which type of exercise you will do depending on what you need in that moment. Each exercise also includes a bonus activity to expand your practice.

The most important thing to remember is to take your time, be kind to yourself, and enjoy the journey!

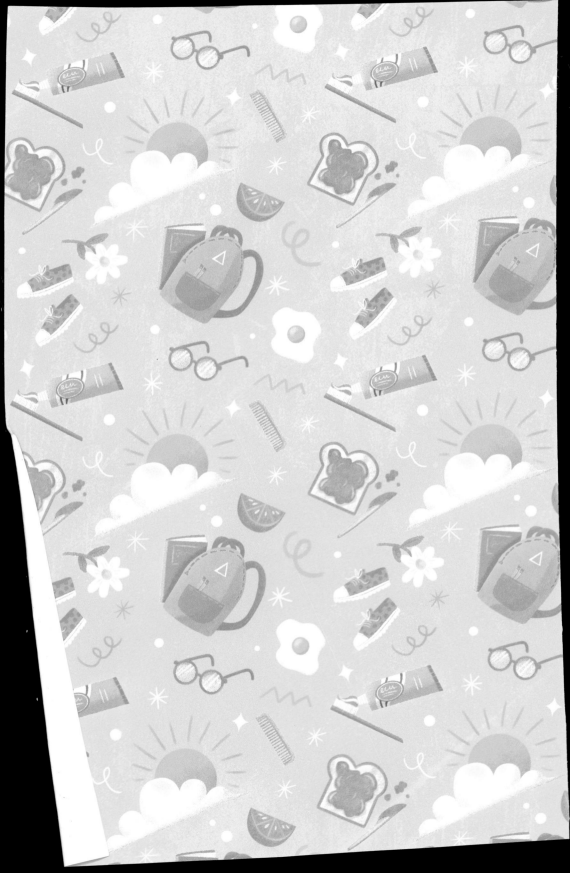

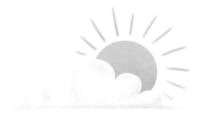

PART ONE

Mindful Mornings

Manic Mornings No More!

Does a typical morning in your home feel rushed? As soon as you wake up for school, you have to get dressed, brush your teeth, comb your hair, pack your backpack, and squeeze in breakfast before you even walk out the front door. Busy mornings like these can cause you to feel worried or anxious. The good news is that you have the power to change these manic mornings by practicing mindfulness. The exercises on the following pages can help you feel calmer, more focused, and more prepared to begin your day—even on Mondays!

EXERCISE 1

GRATEFUL GOOD MORNING

When you wake up in the morning, you may not automatically think positive thoughts. Perhaps you start thinking about the day ahead. Before you know it, your mind is racing before your feet even hit the floor. Have you ever experienced something similar? Imagine what it would be like to start your day on a positive note. Do you think it would change your outlook and maybe the outcome of your day? Try practicing the Grateful Good Morning. It will help fill your mind and heart with grateful thoughts and start your day with good feelings.

1. While you're still in bed, set a timer for 5 minutes.

2. Think of one thing you are grateful for. It can be your family, your home, or something as simple as the warmth of your bed.

3. Keep that image or feeling in your mind as you gently close your eyes and take a deep breath. Breathe in through your nose and then exhale out through your nose.

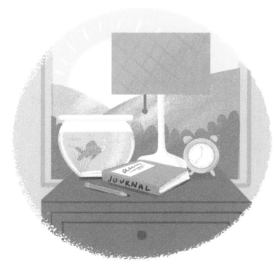

4. With each inhale, say in your mind, "I am grateful."

5. With each exhale, silently say in your mind, "For you."

6. Repeat this until your timer goes off.

7. When you are finished, gently blink your eyes open and begin your day.

WRITE AND REFLECT

Keep a notebook and a pen or pencil next to your bed. Every morning when you wake up, make a note of what you are grateful for. At the end of each week, go back and reflect on everything on your list.

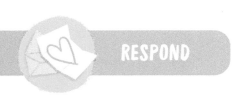
EXERCISE 2

I AM ...

Sometimes we are our own worst critics. That means we say things to ourselves that are not kind. The more negative things we say to ourselves, the more likely we are to believe those things. What do you think would happen if we started speaking kindly to ourselves instead? Sooner or later, we would begin believing those positive things. In this exercise, you will focus on all that is wonderful about you and everything that makes you special. You can practice this any time of day, but it is perfect for mornings. Feeling good about yourself will set you up for a mindful day.

1. Sit comfortably and set a timer for 5 minutes.
2. Gently close your eyes or simply lower your eyelids and allow your eyes to relax.
3. Take a deep breath in through your nose and out through your nose.
4. Think of something you love about

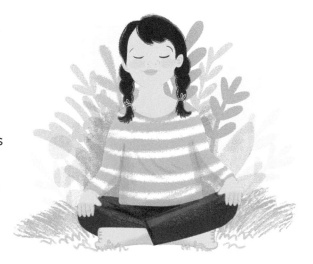

yourself. For example, "I am kind," "I am a good friend," "I am positive," or "I am helpful."

5. Repeat the "I am" statement in your mind as you breathe in and out through your nose.

6. If at any point you feel your mind start to wander, bring it back by focusing on the "I am" statement. Repeat it over and over.

7. When you are finished, gently blink your eyes open.

WRITE AND REFLECT

Write your "I am" statement on a piece of paper or sticky note. Put it somewhere you will see it daily, like on your mirror. Whenever you see the note, repeat your "I am" statement to yourself.

EXERCISE 3

YOU ARE ...

How does it feel when someone says something nice to you? Does it make you feel good? How about when you say something nice to someone else? That feels good, too! Saying kind things to others spreads joy, just as thinking kind thoughts about others creates joy for ourselves. This exercise will show you how to start your day by sending kind wishes to those you love, no matter where they are.

1. Sit comfortably and set a timer for 5 minutes.

2. Gently close your eyes or simply lower your eyelids and allow your eyes to relax.

3. Take a deep breath in through your nose and out through your nose.

4. Picture someone you love. Think of one quality about them that makes them so special. For example, "You are kind," "You are funny," or "You are smart."

5. Repeat the "You are" statement in your mind as you breathe in and out through your nose.

6. If at any point you feel your mind start to wander, bring it back by focusing on the "You are" statement.

7. When you are finished, gently blink your eyes open.

> **WRITE AND REFLECT**
> Think about the person from your "You are" statement. How do you feel when you think about them? Write words to describe your feelings.

EXERCISE 4

BREAKFAST OF CHAMPIONS

Breakfast is an important meal that helps set you up for success each day. Try to make the time to sit down each morning and eat a healthy breakfast. While eating, take a moment for a short gratitude practice and notice how it makes you feel.

1. Sit at the table and set a timer for 10 minutes. Notice how you are feeling.

2. While you eat your breakfast, mentally make a list of things you are grateful for. It could include anything, like your favorite cereal.

3. When the timer goes off, write down your list. Try to see how many things you can remember. If you have a journal or notebook, write the date at the top of the list.

4. When you are finished writing your list, notice how you are feeling. Do you feel happier or calmer than before you started?

5. At the end of each week, go back and read what you wrote. Soon you will have a notebook filled with things that make you grateful and bring you joy.

DID YOU KNOW?

Research has shown that eating a healthy breakfast can help kids focus and concentrate better in class, be more creative, and miss fewer days of school.

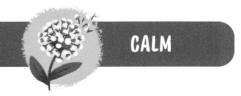

EXERCISE 5

RISE AND SHINE STRETCH

School days can be really rushed. From the moment you wake up, there might be a lot of racing around that continues throughout the day. What you may not realize is that all this rushing makes the muscles in your body super tight. Just like an athlete warming up for a game or race, we also need to warm up our bodies before beginning our day. You can do this before you even get out of bed!

1. While you're still in bed, set a timer for 5 minutes.

2. Gently rock your head from side to side as you lie on your back.

3. Wiggle your fingers and wiggle your toes.

4. Slowly make fists with your hands, then stretch your fingers open wide.

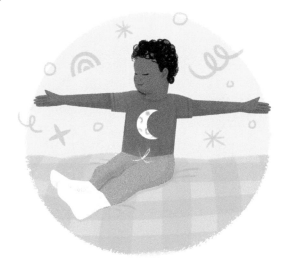

5. Let your ankles roll from side to side.

6. Reach your arms out to the sides as far as you can for a big stretch. As you stretch,

take a deep breath in through your nose and exhale out through your mouth.

7. With your arms stretched, point your toes and reach them toward the end of your bed as far as you can. Take another deep breath in through your nose and exhale out through your mouth.

8. Gently pull your knees in toward your belly. Wrap your arms around your shins and rock from side to side.

9. Roll over onto one side and rise out of bed.

GO DEEPER
Sit up in bed, open your arms wide, and gently turn your upper body from side to side to continue the stretch before getting out of bed.

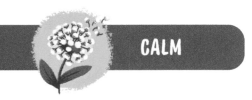

EXERCISE 6

WEEKEND STRETCH

If you enjoyed the weekday Rise and Shine Stretch on page 8, try the extended weekend version. This exercise builds upon the stretches that you practiced during the week with more mindful movement.

1. After you practice the Rise and Shine Stretch, set a timer for 5 minutes.

2. Stand next to your bed with both feet flat on the floor and parallel to each other. Reach your arms out to the sides and overhead as if you are trying to touch the ceiling.

3. Breathe in through your nose and out through your mouth as you reach your fingertips toward the ceiling.

4. On your next inhale, gently lean to your right side with your arms reaching toward the wall to your right.

5. On your exhale, come back up to stand with your arms and hands reaching to the ceiling.

6. On your next inhale, gently lean to your left side with your arms reaching toward the wall to your left.

7. Exhale and bring your body back to center, keeping your fingertips reaching toward the ceiling.

8. Inhale one more time, reaching toward the ceiling. On your exhale, fold forward over your legs with your fingertips reaching toward the floor. Gently let your head hang here and sway your arms from side to side as you continue to inhale and exhale through your nose.

9. On your next inhale, slowly come to stand.

DID YOU KNOW?

When practicing mindful movement, forward-folding poses are calming, cooling poses. Try it whenever you feel you need a break!

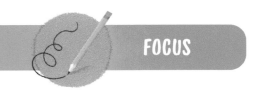

EXERCISE 7

MINDFUL BRUSHING

How many times a day do you brush your teeth? When you brush, how often do you actually think about what you're doing? Are you mindfully brushing or just going through the motions? Practicing mindful brushing can help us reconnect with our senses and clear our minds for the day ahead.

1. Stand at your bathroom sink and set a timer for 5 minutes.

2. Pick up the toothpaste and remove the cap. Then pick up your toothbrush. Gently squeeze the toothpaste onto your toothbrush.

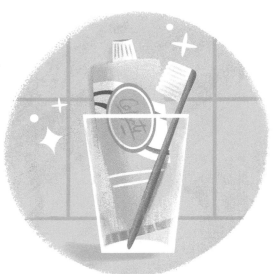

3. Notice how the toothbrush feels in your hand. Is it heavy? Light?

4. Run some water over the toothbrush head before you begin.

5. Can you smell the toothpaste as you bring your toothbrush to your mouth?

6. Begin to brush your teeth. Notice the water you ran over the toothbrush. Is it cold or warm? Notice the toothpaste. What does it taste like?

7. When you finish brushing, rinse your toothbrush under the water.

8. Rinse out your mouth with water. Notice the water in your mouth. How does it feel?

9. Wipe your mouth with a towel and notice the feeling of the towel on your skin.

GO DEEPER

Take a moment to reflect on what you were thinking about while brushing your teeth. Were you able to focus on the brushing? The feel of the bristles? The taste of the toothpaste? Or did your mind wander?

EXERCISE 8

TODAY I WILL ...

Each day gives us a new opportunity to be our best selves, whatever that may be. To be our best, we can set an intention. This is a type of plan for something you are working toward. Intentions can be big things, like "I will get 100 on my math test today," or smaller things, like "I will not make fun of my brother today." An intention should be attainable. That means it is something we are capable of achieving. No matter what your intentions are, each time you set them is a new opportunity for success. Give it a try!

1. Find a pen or pencil and a piece of paper.

2. Sit comfortably and set a timer for 5 minutes.

3. Begin writing a list of intentions. Start each intention with the words: *Today I will.*

4. When the 5 minutes are up, stop writing and pick one intention from the list.

5. Set a timer for another 5 minutes.

6. Gently close your eyes.

7. Silently repeat the intention you chose to yourself as you slowly breathe in and out through your nose.

8. If at any point you feel your mind start to wander, bring it back by focusing on your "Today I will" statement. Repeat it over and over.

9. When you are finished, gently blink your eyes open.

GO DEEPER

Take time to consider that day's intention in more depth. If your intention is to get 100 on your math test, ask yourself why. How will achieving that intention make you feel? What good things will it bring into your life? Carry your thinking forward. If you get 100 on your test today, how will that help you tomorrow? For example, will your good grade make you more motivated to work hard on your homework? How will that help you next week? Next month? Take a deep breath and let it out. Bring your attention back to the present and trust that you can achieve your intention.

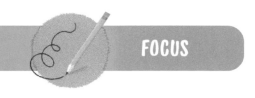

EXERCISE 9

I SPY WITH MY MINDFUL EYE

We often rush through our mornings on autopilot, doing the same thing in the same way. Do you take the same route to school every day? If so, how many times have you passed the same houses without even noticing what color they are? Play this game of I Spy to see how mindful you can be!

1. On your way to school, take a moment to focus on something that you may have never noticed before. For example, a tree, a crack in the sidewalk, or a house.

2. Try to notice the qualities of the thing you are looking at. If it is a tree, what colors do you see? Does the tree have leaves? Are there any animals living in the tree?

3. Every day on your way to school, see if you can discover or notice something new. If you decide to stay focused on one thing, like the tree, try to notice something new about it each day.

> **WRITE AND REFLECT**
>
> Find a time in your day to write about the new thing you noticed. Write down everything you remember about it, no matter how small.

EXERCISE 10

WAKING UP THE SENSES: SIGHT

Just as our bodies wake up each day, so do our senses. Practice paying attention to your senses, beginning with sight. You can awaken your senses whenever you like, but doing it in the morning can help you focus more throughout the day. All you need for this exercise are your eyes.

1. While you are still in bed, set a timer for 8 minutes.

2. Take a moment to let your eyes adjust to the light. Notice the light in your room. Is it bright or dim?

3. Once your eyes have adjusted, look around your room. Try to notice something that you have never noticed before. It may be a spot on the wall or piece of fuzz on the floor.

4. Let your eyes rest gently on that spot.

5. Begin to breathe slowly in and out through your nose.

6. Continue to breathe with your eyes gently focused on that spot.

GO DEEPER

The next time you wake up in the morning, repeat this exercise but add one more minute to your timer.

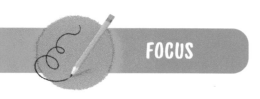

EXERCISE 11

WAKING UP THE SENSES: HEARING

Every day is filled with many different sounds and distractions. This can make it hard to listen when our parents, teachers, or friends are talking. By practicing this exercise, you can strengthen your ability to pay attention and listen mindfully. These focusing skills are really helpful at home and at school. All you need for this exercise are your ears.

1. Sit comfortably and set a timer for 8 minutes.
2. Slowly breathe in and out through your nose. Allow yourself a few moments to settle by focusing only on your breath.
3. Notice the sounds around you. Try to listen for a sound far away from you. Focus on that sound as you continue to breathe in and out through your nose.
4. Next, bring your attention to a sound closer to you. Perhaps it's a sound within your own body. Focus your attention on that sound as you continue to breathe in and out through your nose.
5. Gently open your eyes and let them adjust to the light in the room.

> **GO DEEPER**
>
> Practice this exercise on your way to school by noticing the sounds around you while you are outside. Maybe it's the sound of a bird or a siren in the distance. Take a moment to breathe as you listen to the sound.

EXERCISE 12

WAKING UP THE SENSES: SMELL

What is your favorite smell? Have you ever thought about that? Our sense of smell can bring up memories or experiences we have had, both good and bad. It can also bring our attention to the present moment. For this exercise, practice waking up your sense of smell during breakfast.

1. Sit at the table and set a timer for 10 minutes.
2. Take in all the smells around you. Notice how many different things you can smell.
3. Next, focus on one thing in your breakfast, like a slice of toast or a piece of fruit. Notice the smell of this food. Does it bring up any memories?
4. Notice how the smell makes you feel. Focus on those feelings as you breathe in and out through your nose.

GO DEEPER

Close your eyes the next time you practice this exercise. Does your sense of smell increase? Notice what memories come to mind when you focus on your sense of smell.

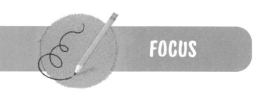
EXERCISE 13

WAKING UP THE SENSES: TASTE

One of the most enjoyable senses to awaken is the sense of taste. Slowing down and eating mindfully helps you truly enjoy and appreciate your food. By eating more slowly and mindfully, we give our bodies time to digest our food. This also gives our minds time to enjoy these foods. You can practice this exercise with any meal, but let's begin with breakfast.

1. Prepare your favorite breakfast.
2. Sit at the table and set a timer for 10 minutes.
3. Slowly take a bite of your food and notice all the different flavors in your mouth.
4. Notice if the food is sweet or savory, hot or cold, soft or hard.
5. Notice how you are chewing your food. If you are chewing quickly, see if you can slow down.
6. Notice what you enjoy about the food you are eating. Think about how this makes you feel.

> **DID YOU KNOW?**
> Chewing your food more slowly before you swallow can help improve your digestion and eliminate stomachaches.

EXERCISE 14

WAKING UP THE SENSES: TOUCH

Do you have a favorite piece of clothing? Maybe it's a T-shirt or a cozy sweater. How about a favorite blanket or stuffed animal? What makes them your favorite? Is it the way they look? Or maybe the way they feel? Touching these things can bring comfort, joy, or happy memories. The sense of touch can activate different areas of our brains that may help us feel more relaxed. Wake up this sense with a simple calming exercise.

1. Sit comfortably and set a timer for 8 minutes.

2. Gently close your eyes.

3. Slowly breathe in and out through your nose.

4. Bring your attention to your feet. Notice how they feel. Are you barefoot? Are you wearing socks or shoes?

5. Wiggle your toes and notice how they feel. Are they cold? Are they warm?

6. Sit for a moment just noticing your feet as you continue to breathe slowly.

7. Gently open your eyes and let them adjust to the light in the room. Notice how you are feeling.

GO DEEPER

Try this exercise again and focus on a different part of your body. Instead of your feet, you could notice your hands. What are they touching? What does it feel like?

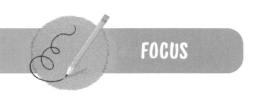
EXERCISE 15

THE FIVE SENSES

Have you ever noticed which of your five senses is strongest? It might depend on what you're doing. If you're listening to music, you're probably focused on hearing. Are you reading a book? Maybe your sense of sight is strongest. Practice using all your senses together in this exercise. Noticing the five senses will help you be present in the moment.

1. Choose a snack (for example, an apple) and set it on a table.

2. Sit comfortably in front of your food. Then set a timer for 10 minutes.

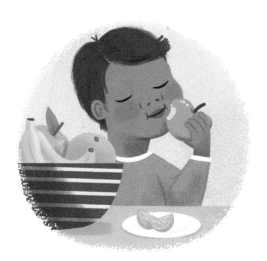

3. Slowly breathe in and out through your nose. Allow yourself a few moments to settle by focusing only on your breath.

4. Look at the food. Notice the colors of your food. How many colors can you see?

5. Pick up your food and notice how it feels in your hand. Is it heavy or light? Is it cold or warm?

6. Smell your food. What does it smell like?

7. Take a bite of your food. What does it taste like? Is it sweet? Is it salty?

8. Finally, notice the sound your chewing makes as you eat. Is it loud in your head? Does it sound muffled?

WRITE AND REFLECT

Which sense is the most important to you? Take a few minutes to write down all the things you appreciate about it. The next time you try this exercise, choose a different sense to write about.

EXERCISE 16

MINDFUL MINUTE

When you are feeling nervous, anxious, excited, tired, happy, or sad, you can practice the Mindful Minute. It's an exercise for any situation you may be in! Focusing on your breath helps clear and calm the mind.

1. Sit comfortably and gently close your mouth.

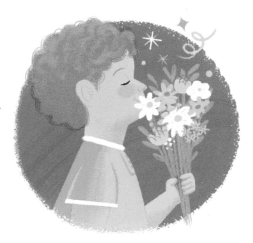

2. Take a deep breath in through your nose. Imagine you have a bouquet of beautiful flowers in front of you. As you inhale deeply, smell those flowers. Breathe out through your nose.

3. Continue to breathe in and out through your nose for three to four breaths.

4. Set a timer for 1 minute.

5. Now begin to count as you breathe, like this:
   - Breathing in through your nose, count silently and slowly: 1, 2.
   - Breathing out through your nose, count silently and slowly: 1, 2, 3, 4.

- Breathing in through your nose, count silently and slowly: 1, 2, 3.

- Breathing out through your nose, count silently and slowly: 1, 2, 3, 4, 5.

6. Continue this pattern of breathing, making each exhale longer than each inhale.

> **GO DEEPER**
>
> At the end of this exercise, notice how you are feeling. Do you feel calmer than you did before you began? Pick a time each day to practice your Mindful Minute. With each practice, add one more minute to your timer.

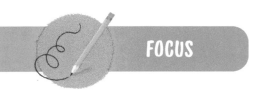

EXERCISE 17

HIGH FIVE BREATHING

This fun exercise will help you bring your attention to the present moment. Try it when you need to be alert and focused on what you are doing. There's no equipment necessary—just use your hands!

1. Sit comfortably and set a timer for 8 minutes.

2. Hold up one hand, fingers spread, with the palm facing away from your body.

3. Place the pointer finger of your other hand at the bottom of your thumb. You're going to use your pointer finger to trace the fingers of the hand you're holding up.

4. Inhale as you trace up your thumb. Then exhale as you trace down your thumb.

5. Inhale as you trace up your pointer finger. Then exhale as you trace down your pointer finger.

6. Continue on tracing each finger until you reach the base of your pinkie finger.

7. Repeat by starting at the base of your pinkie finger. Work your way back to your thumb.

> **GO DEEPER**
>
> Try doing this exercise with the opposite hand. If you started by tracing your left hand with your right pointer finger, switch it up by tracing your right hand with your left pointer finger!

EXERCISE 18

DO YOU HEAR WHAT I HEAR?

There is a famous saying that goes, "The quieter you become, the more you hear." This means that the more we quiet ourselves and our minds, the more present we will become. By tuning in to the sounds around you, you will be able to focus your mind and your body for the day ahead.

1. While you are sitting or lying on your bed, set a timer for 8 minutes.

2. Take a moment to listen to the sounds around you.

3. Gently close your mouth and take a deep breath in through your nose. Then exhale out through your nose.

4. Notice all the sounds you can hear. Bring your attention to the sound that is farthest from you, such as birds chirping or cars going by.

5. Bring your attention to the sound that is closest to you. Continue to inhale and exhale through your nose as you focus on the sound.

> **GO DEEPER**
> Practice this mindful listening exercise throughout the day and notice what sounds bring you joy. Do you have a favorite sound? How does it make you feel?

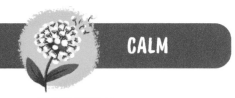

EXERCISE 19

BUS STOP BREATHING

One of the best things about mindfulness is that you can practice it anywhere and at any time. If you take a bus to school, you can do this breathing exercise while you wait for the bus to arrive. You can even do it on the bus (or in the car if someone drives you to school). This exercise helps calm your nerves and clear your mind for the school day ahead.

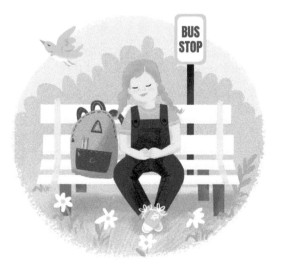

1. When you arrive at the bus stop, set a timer for 3 minutes.

2. Bring your attention to your breath. Slowly inhale and exhale through your nose.

3. With each inhale, notice how your belly expands, or grows larger, as you breathe in.

4. With each exhale, notice how your belly collapses, or gets smaller, as you exhale.

5. Continue to breathe slowly while noticing the movement of your belly.

6. If at any time during your practice you notice your mind start to wander, that's okay! Just bring your attention back to your breath once again.

7. When you are finished, notice how you are feeling.

DID YOU KNOW?

Practicing mindful breathing can help calm your nervous system and focus your mind. It's a great way to start your day!

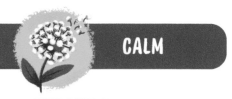

EXERCISE 20

MORNING MOVEMENT

Have you ever noticed that the more you rush, the more things seem to go wrong? You know those mornings: You are late for school, so you hurry to the door, only to trip on the way and spill everything out of your backpack. What do you think would happen if we slowed down instead? Even when things seem rushed, you can take your time and move with mindfulness. There is no need to time this exercise because you will do it throughout your morning.

1. Before getting up out of bed, take a moment to listen to the sounds around you. Notice what you hear. Can you hear sounds outside your room? How about outside your house?

2. While listening to the sounds around you, take a deep breath in through your nose and exhale out through your nose.

3. As you slowly get out of bed, notice your feet the moment they touch the floor. Is the floor cold? Warm? Notice each of your toes on the floor.

4. Take a moment to stand at the edge of your bed, breathing in and out through your nose.

5. As you slowly get dressed, notice the feel of your clothing as it touches your skin.

6. Take your time as you walk toward the breakfast table and sit down. Notice how this morning may feel different from a morning when you were rushing.

7. Continue to move mindfully as you go through your morning routine. Anytime you start to feel rushed throughout your day, such as when you're hurrying from one class to the next, try to come back to this sense of mindful movement.

WRITE AND REFLECT

How does it feel to take your time in the morning as you start your day? Does slowly rising from bed and taking a few deep breaths help set up your day for success? Write about how mindfully moving through your morning was or wasn't helpful to you.

Life is a dance.
Mindfulness is witnessing
that dance.

—Amit Ray

PART TWO

Midday Mindfulness

What Are Your Days Like?

Our days can be filled with lots of activity and many expectations. Expectations are things we place on ourselves, but there are also expectations that others have of us. All of this makes us experience different emotions throughout each day. Some emotions feel good, like joy, happiness, and gratitude. Other emotions might not feel so good, like anger, frustration, and anxiety. When we practice mindfulness, we train our brains to become more aware of all these different emotions. This helps us respond to them in a positive way.

The more you practice being mindful, the quicker your brain will learn how to respond in all kinds of situations. Pretty cool, right? The exercises in this section can help reenergize your mind and body in the middle of the day. There are also exercises to calm you after a hectic school day when you need time to yourself.

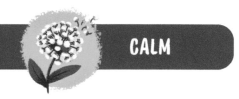

EXERCISE 21

BELL BREATHING

Most weekdays are filled with school bells that ring numerous times throughout your day. Sometimes the bell can surprise or startle you if you weren't expecting it. This reaction is known as our "fight or flight" response. It is your body's way of reacting to a perceived threat. You can learn to react in a calmer way through mindfulness. Use the opportunity of bells ringing throughout the day as a reminder to take some mindful breaths.

1. Every time you hear the school bell, take a slow, deep breath in through your nose and out through your nose.
2. Continue to breathe slowly as you move through your school after the bell rings.
3. Notice how you feel.

> **GO DEEPER**
>
> Use this same exercise for any sound that startles you, such as a car horn, a text alert, or a ringing phone.

EXERCISE 22

NOTICE THE PAUSE

Mindfulness can help us respond to situations instead of reacting to them. This is sometimes known as learning to "notice the pause." The pause is that moment or space between something happening and your response or reaction to it. Practice this exercise to begin noticing the pause.

1. The next time you find yourself in a situation where your first reaction might be to get mad or upset, pause.

2. Notice how you feel when you pause. Notice where you feel this feeling in your body. How does it feel?

3. Once you have identified the feeling, take a few deep breaths in and out through your nose.

4. Notice how you are feeling now. Can you respond to the situation in a more mindful way?

DID YOU KNOW?

When you take a moment to breathe before reacting, you begin to train your brain. You learn to think before speaking or acting on your immediate impulses. The more you practice this, the more you will notice the pause in every situation.

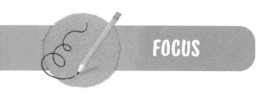

EXERCISE 23

TRAIN YOUR BRAIN

In gym class, you exercise your body to keep it strong. You can also exercise your brain to keep it strong, calm, and focused. By practicing mindfulness, you can train your brain to make good choices and pay attention in school and at home.

1. Set a timer for 8 minutes.
2. Stand up tall with your feet hip-width apart. Keep your arms down by your sides.
3. Take a deep breath in through your nose, then exhale out through your nose.
4. On your next inhale, sweep your arms out from your sides and reach them overhead so your palms meet above.
5. On your next exhale, bring your arms all the way back down by your sides.
6. Continue breathing in and out through your nose while sweeping your arms from your sides to over your head.

GO DEEPER

The next time you do this exercise, try folding forward over your legs as you exhale. Sweep your arms over your head and reach your hands toward the floor. When you inhale, reach up overhead. Then repeat the forward fold on the exhale.

CALM

EXERCISE 24

MINDFUL REMINDER

How many text messages, emails, or other notifications do you receive? There is a lot of information that comes at us all day, every day. Sometimes it can feel like too much, right? Instead of looking at your screen every time you receive a message alert, take a few moments to breathe. In this exercise, you will use the message alert sound on your phone or device as a reminder to practice mindfulness. What do you think will happen?

1. Each time you receive an alert, take a moment to resist the urge to check your phone or device.

2. Instead, close your eyes and take a deep breath in through your nose and exhale out through your nose.

3. If you find this difficult, consider changing your notification settings so that you receive phone alerts less often. When you think about checking your phone, follow the step above to practice mindful breathing instead.

GO DEEPER

Continue this practice all afternoon and evening. At bedtime, reflect on how it felt to look at your phone less often.

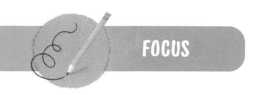
EXERCISE 25

MINDFUL WALKING

School days can be hectic. Bells ring loudly, doors fly open, and hallways are crowded with students. You can give yourself a break and slow down even when things are busy. Practice mindful walking throughout your day with this exercise.

1. Find somewhere safe to practice mindful walking, like your yard, a park, or inside your house.

2. Set a timer for 10 minutes.

3. Stand still and bring your attention to your breath.

4. Breathe slowly and deeply, inhaling and exhaling through your nose.

5. Start walking slowly. When you practice mindful walking, the goal is not to reach any specific destination. The goal is to notice how you feel during the walk.

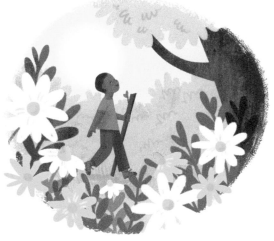

6. Notice how your feet feel with each step. Which part of your foot touches the ground first when you take a step?

7. Notice how your body feels. Does it feel heavy or light today?

8. Notice the way you walk. Are you slouching? Or are you standing up straight? Try not to change the way you walk. Instead, just notice how your body naturally moves.

9. Continue to breathe deeply in and out through your nose as you walk.

10. If at any point your mind starts to wander, simply bring it back to your breath and focus on each step.

11. When the timer stops, notice how you are feeling.

DID YOU KNOW?

Walking has many benefits. It can improve our mood, lower stress, lower blood pressure, and help us sleep better. Mindful walking can also create feelings of happiness.

EXERCISE 26

MASTER THE EMOTION-COASTER

Our emotions or feelings can change moment by moment. There are many things that may affect your emotions throughout the day. You might have nerves over an upcoming test or presentation, an argument with a friend, or problems at home with your family. Sometimes our changing emotions may feel like we are riding a roller coaster with many highs and just as many lows. Practicing mindfulness can help us learn how to ride the coaster with more calm and ease. This exercise can help teach us how to master the emotion-coaster.

1. Sit comfortably and set a timer for 8 minutes.

2. Gently close your eyes. Remember a time when you felt like your emotions were high, like when you felt nervous, anxious, or angry.

3. Notice how it feels in your body when you remember these emotions. Do you feel any sensations in your body when remembering?

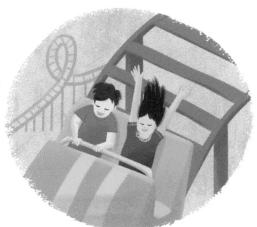

4. Bring your attention to any areas of the body where you feel sensations.

5. Slowly breathe in through your nose. As you inhale, imagine you are heading up to the tall peak of a roller coaster. Continue to inhale until you reach the peak.

6. At the peak of the roller coaster, hold your breath.

7. Exhale all the air out through your nose, imagining the roller coaster heading down from the peak. Extend your exhale to make it longer than your inhale.

8. Repeat this breathing pattern until your timer goes off.

DID YOU KNOW?

When you inhale, your heartbeat speeds up. When you exhale, your heartbeat slows down. Practicing a longer exhale will help calm your body and mind.

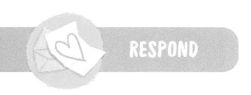

EXERCISE 27

POSITIVE PINKIE WORDS

The way you think about something affects the way you feel about it. For example, if you keep telling yourself that you are nervous about a test, it will make you more nervous about the test! What do you think would happen if you replaced the word "nervous" with a positive word? Instead of saying, "I am so nervous," you could say, "I am so prepared." Try it by practicing positive pinkie words.

1. Sit comfortably and set a timer for 8 minutes.

2. Place your hands on your knees with your palms facing up.

3. Touch your thumb to your pointer finger and say, "I."

4. Touch your thumb to your middle finger and say, "Am."

5. Touch your thumb to your ring finger and say, "So."

6. Touch your thumb to your pinkie and say "Calm." This pinkie word can be replaced by any other word that may help in that moment: *relaxed*, *happy*, *smart*, *prepared*, *ready*.

7. Start back at the beginning with your thumb to your pointer finger and slowly repeat these words over and over.

> **DID YOU KNOW?**
> Saying a statement repeatedly is called a *mantra*. Practicing a mantra can reduce anxiety.

EXERCISE 28

THOUGHT TRAIN

There are many ways to practice mindful breathing; however, it does not make the thoughts in our minds stop. Our minds are always thinking. In fact, you probably have thousands of thoughts per day! Practicing mindful breathing can help you notice when a new thought pops into your head. By noticing those thoughts and when they wander, you are being mindful. In this exercise, you will notice a thought but then let it continue to move on, like a train.

1. Sit comfortably and set a timer for 5 minutes.

2. Begin breathing in and out through your nose.

3. Focus your attention on your breathing. When you breathe in, say "inhale" in your mind. When you breathe out, say "exhale" in your mind.

4. When a thought pops into your mind, simply bring your attention back to your focus words: *inhale* and *exhale*.

5. Continue breathing this way until your timer goes off.

6. Notice how you are feeling.

> **GO DEEPER**
>
> Add one more minute to your timer the next time you practice this exercise. See if you can get to 10 minutes of mindful breathing with fewer thoughts distracting you.

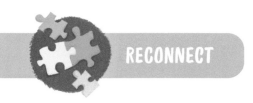

EXERCISE 29

MY WISH FOR YOU

Sending kind wishes to those we care about is a wonderful way to spread kindness and love. But we can also send kind wishes to those we don't get along with and those we don't know well. When we send kind wishes to others, it can help us feel good, too.

1. Sit comfortably and set a timer for 8 minutes.

2. Close your eyes and begin to breathe slowly in and out through your nose.

3. Allow yourself to settle into your breathing for a few moments. When you are ready, picture in your mind someone you may not get along with or someone you do not know well. It could be a person who may have hurt your feelings. See this person clearly in your mind.

4. As you think of this person, repeat these words in your mind:

May you be happy.
May you be healthy.
May you be peaceful.
May you be loved.

> **GO DEEPER**
> Practice sending kind wishes to yourself by repeating the same words as above but replacing the "you" with "I." Say to yourself, "May I be happy. May I be healthy. May I be peaceful. May I be loved."

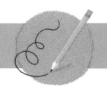

EXERCISE 30

INFINITY BREATHING

The average person takes 12 to 18 breaths per minute. But when we are anxious, nervous, or upset, we begin to breathe much faster. Try this experiment to see how many breaths per minute you usually take. Then see if you can focus on your breath and notice how it makes you feel.

1. Sit comfortably on the floor and set a timer for 1 minute.

2. Count how many breaths you take during this minute. This is your normal rate of breathing.

3. Next, set a timer for 6 minutes.

4. Touch the floor with your pointer finger. Imagine that you are touching the center of the number 8. Slowly trace your finger around the left side of the 8 while breathing in.

5. When you return to the center, trace your finger around the right side as you slowly breathe out.

6. Continue tracing until the timer goes off.

7. Notice if you were breathing faster or more slowly than when you started.

> **GO DEEPER**
>
> Practice tracing the 8 in reverse order. Begin with your finger in the center of the 8. Go up and around the right side this time.

CALM

SHRUG IT OFF

Do you ever notice how often you are looking down? You probably spend a lot of time hunched over a desk or computer at school. And that probably continues at home when doing your homework or using a phone. When you spend so much time looking down, you put a lot of pressure and stress on your neck and shoulders. It's a good idea to take some time throughout the day to bring our attention to that part of our bodies. When you feel like you need a break at any time during the day, do this exercise to shrug it off.

1. Set a timer for 8 minutes.
2. You can practice this exercise in a seated position or standing tall with your feet hip-width apart, knees slightly bent, arms down by your sides, and palms facing away from your body.
3. Slowly breathe in. As you inhale, shrug like you are trying to touch your shoulders to your earlobes.
4. Hold your breath as you count to 10 in your mind.

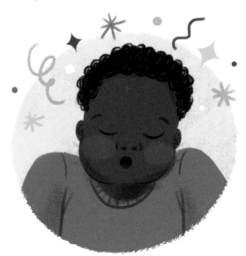

5. Drop your shoulders away from your ears as you exhale loudly, making a "huh" sound.

6. Repeat until the timer goes off.

DID YOU KNOW?

You can set up the space where you do your homework to help prevent tension from building in your neck and back. Adjust your chair or where you place your laptop or computer monitor so your eyes are level with the top of the screen. Adjust the height of your chair or, if you can, your desk or table so that your forearms are parallel to the floor. Keep any items you need to use often, like your computer mouse, your pen or pencil, or your schoolbooks, in easy reach, so you can stay sitting tall as you work.

EXERCISE 32

RAINBOW ENERGY

Your energy usually ranges between high and low through-out the day. Sometimes you feel super energized and ready to go, like on the playground during recess or when you move around in gym class. There are also times when your energy is low. You might feel this after lunch or during a long class. If you want to increase your energy and give yourself a boost, try this simple breathing exercise!

1. Set a timer for 3 minutes.

2. Stand tall with your feet hip-width apart, knees slightly bent, arms down by your sides, and palms facing away from your body.

3. As you inhale, sweep your arms out to the sides. Reach your arms overhead so your palms touch above.

4. As you exhale, release your arms back down by your sides.

5. On your next inhale, picture your favorite color of the rainbow. As you sweep your arms out to meet overhead, imagine surrounding your entire body with that color.

6. As you exhale, release your arms back down by your sides and imagine your favorite color pouring down on your body.

7. Repeat, imagining different colors of the rainbow, until the timer goes off.

> **GO DEEPER**
>
> After the timer goes off, stand with your eyes closed and notice how you feel. Then practice the exercise again with your eyes closed. Notice if the practice is harder or easier.

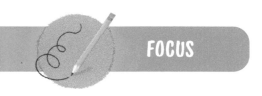

EXERCISE 33

FEET ON THE GROUND

There may be times when you feel like everything in your life is moving way too fast: school, tests, homework, sports, rehearsals, drama with friends. When there is a lot going on around you, it may feel like it's hard to focus or think clearly. Sometimes we just need to take a moment to stop and steady ourselves. You can do this by bringing attention to your feet on the ground. Let's try it!

1. Set a timer for 5 minutes.
2. Stand tall with your feet hip-width apart, knees slightly bent, arms down by your sides, and palms facing away from your body.
3. Notice the feeling of your feet on the ground.
4. Bring your attention to the big toe on each foot. Feel your big toes pressing down on the ground.
5. Bring your attention to the second toe on each foot. Feel these toes pressing down on the ground.
6. Continue until you reach your pinkie toes.
7. When you are finished, notice how you're feeling. Do you feel steadier than when you began?

> **WRITE AND REFLECT**
> Write about a time when you felt like things were out of control. Notice your feelings as you remember this experience. Then, practice the Feet on the Ground exercise. Do you feel calmer or steadier afterward?

EXERCISE 34

A MINDFUL BREAK

After a long day at school, you might not want to come home, sit down, and do homework. Studying at home is a time that can be filled with anxiety, frustration, and melt-downs for a lot of kids. Before you sit down to do your homework, try taking a mindful break. This can help clear your mind, focus your brain, and reduce any stress you may be feeling before you get started.

1. Sit comfortably or lie on the floor. Set a timer for 8 minutes.

2. Count to three in your mind as you take a deep breath in through your nose.

3. Hold that breath as you count to three.

4. Count to three as you slowly exhale.

5. Hold your breath for a count of three.

6. You can use your fingers to keep track as you count. If at any point you lose count, simply start at the beginning.

7. Continue breathing and counting this way until your timer goes off.

GO DEEPER

Each time you come back to practice this exercise, try increasing your counts by one. Start counting to three on Mondays, then count to four on Tuesdays, and so on until Friday.

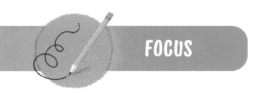
EXERCISE 35

MY MINDFUL ANCHOR

Just like an anchor helps keep a boat steady, our breath helps keep us steady. Think about it: What would happen to the boat if it did not have its anchor? Without anything to hold it in place, maybe the boat would drift away. Our minds can drift away like this, too. But when we learn to use breathing as our anchor, we can focus our attention to steady our minds and bodies.

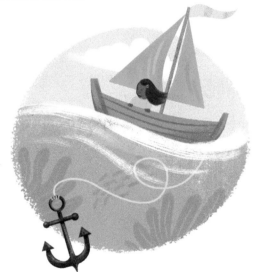

1. Sit comfortably and set a timer for 10 minutes.

2. Breathing normally, notice where in your body you feel your breath the most.

3. Place one hand on your belly. Take a breath to see if you notice your breath in your belly.

4. Place one hand on your chest. Take a breath to see if you notice your breath in your chest.

5. Place one hand on your throat. Take a breath and see if you notice your breath in your throat.

6. Finally, place a finger under your nose and take a breath. Notice the air as it reaches your finger. Is the air warm or cool?

7. Notice where you felt your breath the most. Wherever you feel your breath the most is your "anchor spot." This is the place in your body that is your anchor. Practice breathing into this spot to keep you steady and focused.

WRITE AND REFLECT

Your anchor can change from day to day. For example, you may feel your breath more in your belly on some days, while other days you feel it more in your chest. Write a journal entry each time you practice this exercise to note where you found your anchor that day.

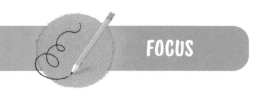

EXERCISE 36

BALANCE AND FOCUS

Do you ever feel tired or sluggish in the middle of the day? This is common for a lot of kids. One thing you can do to fight tiredness is to practice this exercise. Practicing balancing exercises will help focus your mind and energize your body for the rest of the day.

1. Set a timer for 8 minutes.
2. Stand tall with your feet hip-width apart, knees slightly bent, arms down by your sides, and palms facing away from your body.
3. Look at one point or object in front of you. Keep your eyes focused on this point as you breathe in and out through your nose.
4. Balance on your left foot. Bend your right knee and place your right foot on your right calf, or high up on your inner right thigh. Place your hands on your hips.
5. Keep your gaze on your focal point and continue to breathe for five breaths.
6. Come back to your standing pose and repeat on the other side.

> **GO DEEPER**
>
> The next time you do this exercise, try raising your arms straight up overhead as you balance on one foot. Bring the palms of your hands to touch overhead. Take five breaths. To challenge yourself, close your eyes in this pose.

EXERCISE 37

FOCUSING YOUR ZOOM LENS

Sometimes when we are upset or worried about something, we think about it repeatedly. It's like we are hitting a replay button in our minds. When we do this, it's almost as if we are putting our worries under a zoom lens. This makes them appear much larger than they are. You can practice refocusing your zoom lens to bring yourself and your worries into focus. Try this exercise to bring yourself back to the present moment.

1. When you wake up in the morning, pick an object to be your focal point. Make it something that you will have with you all day, like a button on your shirt.

2. Whenever you feel your zoom lens kicking in throughout the day, place your hand on your focal object. Then take a deep breath in and out through your nose.

3. Each time you take a breath, imagine your worry becoming smaller and smaller, as if you are readjusting your lens. Keep adjusting that lens until your worry disappears.

> **GO DEEPER**
> You can also use your zoom lens to emphasize something positive. Touch your focal point to remind yourself of something that makes you happy.

EXERCISE 38

POSITIVE AFFIRMATIONS

There are times when you may feel unsure of yourself. Maybe you are afraid to try something new because you think you will fail or embarrass yourself. Guess what? Everyone has felt this way at one point or another. The way we speak to ourselves in our heads can play a big part in this fear. When you try something new, maybe your head tells you that you cannot do it. It might even tell you that your friend or classmate can do it better. Practicing mindfulness can turn these negative thoughts into positive thoughts called *affirmations*. The more you practice affirmations, the more you can retrain your brain to think positively.

1. Sit comfortably and set a timer for 8 minutes.
2. Focus on your breath as you inhale and exhale through your nose.
3. Notice the thoughts that enter your mind. Notice if these thoughts are negative or positive.
4. When you notice a negative thought, replace it with a positive affirmation. For example, if you have a math test coming up and you are thinking, "Math is too hard and I can't do it," replace that thought with "I can do hard things." Keep your affirmations short and in the present tense by saying things like "I can" and "I will."

5. Inhale as you repeat your affirmation to yourself.

6. Exhale out any negativity that stands in the way of you believing in your affirmation.

7. Continue this cycle until the timer goes off. If you still feel the tension of negative thoughts, continue until you feel it lighten.

GO DEEPER

The more you repeat your positive affirmations, the more you will boost your self-confidence. Write your positive affirmations on sticky notes and place them on your mirror at home, or in your locker at school. Every time you see the sticky notes, take a deep breath and repeat those affirmations to yourself.

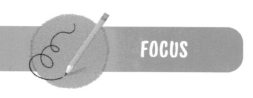

EXERCISE 39

SPINNING TO STILLNESS

Have you ever been on a ride at an amusement park that spins and spins? Everything moves so quickly around you and it feels like it's never going to stop. Sometimes life can feel this way, too. Between school, homework, sports, activities, friends, and family, life just spins and spins. This feeling is totally normal and happens to most people. But guess what? By practicing mindfulness and using the tools you've learned, you can help turn this spinning into stillness. Mindfulness can help us notice our senses so we can steady ourselves in the present moment.

1. Sit comfortably and set a timer for 10 minutes.

2. Look around and notice five things you can see. List those things in your mind.

3. Notice five things you can hear. List those things in your mind.

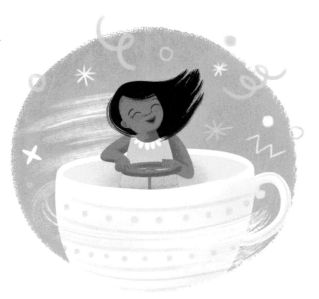

4. Notice five things you can touch and feel. List those things in your mind.

5. Add one more thing you can see to your mental list. Repeat with one more thing you can hear and one more thing you can feel and touch. Continue until your timer goes off.

GO DEEPER

Over the next few days, notice when you start to feel overwhelmed. Notice where you feel it in your body. Maybe you feel butterflies in your stomach, or maybe your heart starts beating faster. Practice the Spinning to Stillness exercise and notice how you feel. Did the exercise bring your mind to stillness?

EXERCISE 40

LOST AND FOUND

Have you ever lost something that was very valuable to you? Or thought you lost something? Maybe it was your phone, a homework assignment, or a favorite toy. The sudden worry or fear you feel can overtake you in an instant. Where in your body do you feel that worry or fear? Can you find it? What does it feel like? Maybe you feel your heart start to race or your hands get sweaty. When you learn to bring your attention to those feelings, you can learn to notice them and label them without judgment. This is mindfulness. Practice this exercise to find those feelings or emotions.

1. The next time you feel worried, anxious, or scared, take a moment to notice your feeling.

2. Notice why you are feeling this way. Is it because of something that happened? Something you are scared might happen? Or is it something more general that has been worrying you, like a difficult class or tension with a friend?

3. Notice how these feelings are making you feel in your body. Is it an actual sensation in some part of your body, like butterflies in your stomach? Is it an overall feeling, like sweating? Just notice.

4. Focus on where you are feeling these sensations.

5. Take a deep breath in through your nose and exhale out through your mouth with a great big sigh. As you exhale, allow the part of your body you are focusing on to relax. Take a moment to feel the ease of tension before repeating.

6. Continue to breathe this way until your body begins to feel calmer.

GO DEEPER

Practice breathing in through your nose and out through your mouth, making a "whoosh" sound every time you exhale. Try to make each exhale longer than each inhale. This lets you release more air at once, which can help reduce anxiety.

Feelings come and
go like clouds in a windy
sky. Conscious breathing
is my anchor.

—Thich Nhat Hanh

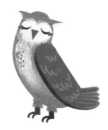

PART THREE

Mindfulness at Night

Breathe into Stillness

At the end of a long day, you are exhausted and ready for bed. But then you get into bed, and what happens? You can't fall asleep! Maybe you have too many thoughts running through your head. Your mind replays the day you had or anticipates what you have coming up tomorrow. It all keeps playing over and over in your head like a movie. The good news is that mindfulness can help calm our minds and bodies at nighttime, not just in the morning and the middle of the day. Practicing mindful movement or mindful meditation before bedtime is a great way to set yourself up for a restful night's sleep.

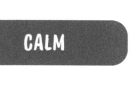
EXERCISE 41

PAUSE BUTTON

Wouldn't it be great if life had a pause button? You could press it whenever you needed a break at school, home, sports, anywhere. But guess what? You *do* have a pause button! It's your breath. You can access it whenever you need a break. It's especially helpful to access your pause button at night. It can help put to rest anything that may have happened during the day and prepare your body for sleep.

1. Sit comfortably and set a timer for 5 minutes.

2. Take a deep breath in through your nose and exhale out through your nose.

3. In your mind, picture a giant button with the word *PAUSE* on it. Continue to imagine your pause button until you can see it clearly. What color is it? How big is it? Does it sparkle or glow?

4. Take a moment to notice any uncomfortable feelings that might have built up during the day, such as worries or concerns about things that have happened or might happen later.

5. Breathe in as you imagine placing your finger on the button. Breathe out as you imagine pressing down on the button. Imagine everything around you has paused, as if frozen in time.

6. Continue to breathe at your own pace.

7. If you feel your mind start to wander, imagine your giant button again. Reach for the button on your next inhale, then press the button and pause everything around you when you exhale.

GO DEEPER

Practice using your pause button whenever you feel like you need a moment to collect your thoughts or reset your mind. To ground yourself, place both hands gently on your belly as you practice.

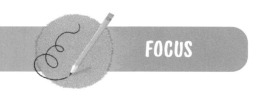

EXERCISE 42

OWL EYES

When you focus your attention on just one thing, you can begin calming your body and mind. This brings you to the present moment. Your focus is like an owl's binocular vision. Like an owl, you can zoom in on something specific. When you do this, it will help all other distractions fade away. Train your brain to stay in the present moment and focus with this exercise.

1. Choose a small object to focus on, such as a toy.
2. Set a timer for 5 minutes.
3. Sit comfortably and close your eyes.
4. Begin your mindful breathing by inhaling and exhaling through your nose.
5. Once your body feels settled, slowly open your eyes. Bring them to rest on the object you chose.
6. Notice the object. Is it colorful? If so, what colors does it have? Is it small or large? Hard or soft? Keep your eyes on the object and just observe.
7. Close your eyes and continue inhaling and exhaling through your nose.

DID YOU KNOW?

This single-focus exercise is a type of meditation. It is a great way for beginners to practice mindfulness. A lot of people find it easier to practice meditation when they have something to focus on or look at.

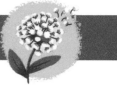

EXERCISE 43

TAP IT OUT

Sleep is really important because it gives your body an opportunity to rest, grow, heal, or fight off illnesses. But sometimes it's not that easy to settle down at the end of the day. One way you can help your body and mind relax is by practicing tapping. When we do this, we can relax different areas of our body just by using our fingers. Check it out!

1. Sit comfortably and set a timer for 8 minutes.

2. Gently tap the top of your head using the fingertips of both hands. Continue tapping as you inhale and exhale three times.

3. Move your fingertips to the area above your eyebrows. Tap as you inhale and exhale three times.

4. Move your fingertips to your temples. Tap as you inhale and exhale three times.

5. Move your fingertips to the area below your jawbone. Tap as you inhale and exhale three times.

6. Move your fingertips to your collarbone. Tap as you inhale and exhale three times.

7. When you are finished, rest your hands down by your sides and notice how you are feeling.

> **DID YOU KNOW?**
> During sleep, your body makes a hormone that helps you grow and helps your body repair muscles and bone.

EXERCISE 44

BODY SCAN

Focusing on different areas of the body helps us relax and prepare for sleep. One way to do this is by practicing a mindful meditation known as the body scan. In this exercise, you will bring all your attention to a particular part of the body and notice any sensations you may feel.

1. Lie comfortably and set a timer for 10 minutes.
2. Close your eyes and begin breathing slowly in and out through your nose.
3. Take a moment to notice any tightness in your body. Simply notice without trying to change it as you breathe slowly in and out through your nose.
4. Bring your attention to the very top of your head. Notice any sensations you may feel at the top of your head.
5. Bring your attention to your face: your forehead, eyes, nose, cheeks, mouth, and chin. Notice any sensations you may feel in your face.
6. Bring your attention to your neck. Notice any sensations you may feel in your neck.
7. Bring your attention to your shoulders. Notice any sensations you may feel in your shoulders.
8. Bring your attention to your arms: your upper arms, elbows, lower arms, and wrists. Notice any sensations you may feel in your arms.

9. Bring your attention to your hands: your thumbs, fingers, and palms. Notice any sensations you may feel in your hands.

10. Bring your attention to your torso: your chest, ribs, and belly. Notice any sensations you may feel in your torso.

11. Bring your attention to your legs: your thighs, knees, calves, and ankles. Notice any sensations you may feel in your legs.

12. Bring your attention to your feet: your toes, heels, the tops of your feet, and the soles of your feet. Notice any sensations you may feel in your feet.

13. Take your time as you scan your body, pausing for a few deep breaths at each point.

14. Notice how you feel.

GO DEEPER

Practice your body scan again. This time, see if you can add another part of your body to the scan. For example, when bringing your attention to your face, notice your tongue. Is it relaxed or is it touching the roof of your mouth? Relax your tongue.

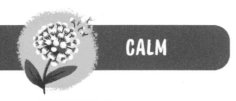

EXERCISE 45

SQUEEZE IT OUT

When you focus on the different parts of your body, you learn to notice any sensations or tensions you may feel in those areas. Practice letting those tensions go by squeezing them out.

1. Lie comfortably and set a timer for 8 minutes.

2. Close your eyes and breathe slowly in and out through your nose.

3. Bring your attention to your toes. Squeeze your toes as tight as you can, then relax your toes. Let your feet gently flop out to each side.

4. Bring your attention to your legs. Squeeze the muscles of your legs as tight as you can, then relax your legs.

5. Bring your attention to your belly. Squeeze the muscles of your belly as tight as you can, then relax your belly.

6. Bring your attention to your fingers. Squeeze your fingers as tight as you can, making two fists with your hands. Then relax each hand and let your fingers fall open.

7. Bring your attention to your shoulders. Shrug your shoulders up as high as you can, as if you are trying to touch your ears with the tops of your shoulders. Release your shoulders away from your ears and exhale a big "Ha!" out through your mouth.

8. Bring your attention to your face. Squeeze all the muscles of your face as tight as you can, then relax your face.

9. Finally, bring your attention to your entire body, from your feet all the way to your head. Squeeze your body as tight as you can, then relax your entire body.

DID YOU KNOW?

This type of body scan is called "progressive muscle relaxation." It's great for relieving stress and anxiety, especially if you practice it regularly. You can use it when you're feeling stressed or when you're feeling calm. The more comfortable you get with it, the more effective it will be at helping you relax.

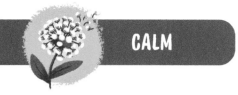

EXERCISE 46

LEGS UP THE WALL

A nighttime routine can help ensure a good night's sleep. This routine could include preparing for the next day by laying out your school clothes and packing your backpack. Another routine is preparing for bed by taking a bath or shower and brushing your teeth. And, of course, practicing mindfulness can be a nighttime routine! This exercise is perfect to add to your routine because it relaxes your muscles and calms your nervous system.

1. Set a timer for 8 minutes.

2. Sit with the right side of your body pressed against a wall.

3. Bend your knees in toward your belly. Then turn your upper body away from the wall. As you turn, extend your legs up the wall and come to lie down on your back. Your legs may be straight, or you can have a slight bend in your knees. Do whatever is most comfortable for you.

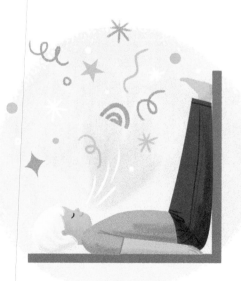

4. Let your arms rest down by your sides and close your eyes.

5. Breathe deeply in and out through your nose.

DID YOU KNOW?

The legs up the wall pose is known to have a variety of benefits, like improving sleep patterns, decreasing stress, gently stretching your muscles, and even things like improving circulation and getting rid of headaches. It's a good pose to use to settle down at night, but you can also use it in the morning or afternoon to help you feel calmer and have more energy.

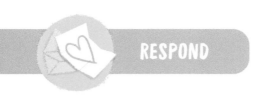
EXERCISE 47

CLOUD MEDITATION

Have you ever laid on the grass outside and watched the clouds float by? Some days they appear to be moving quickly, while other days they look perfectly still. Our thoughts and worries can be like that as well. Sometimes they race by and other times they get stuck in place. Try this short meditation to see if you can clear your mind.

1. Sit comfortably and set a timer for 5 minutes.

2. Close your eyes and take a deep breath in through your nose. Then exhale out through your nose.

3. In your mind, picture a bright blue sky. Imagine big, white, fluffy clouds moving slowly through the sky from left to right.

4. As you watch the clouds float by, think of any worries you may have had throughout the day.

5. Imagine placing your worries softly on the clouds. Watch them float away.

6. As each new worry comes to mind, place it on another cloud and watch it float away with the others.

WRITE AND REFLECT

Draw a picture of clouds in the sky. Write one of your worries on each cloud. If you like, you can make big clouds for your biggest worries and small clouds for your smallest worries. As you write your worries, imagine them floating away on the clouds.

EXERCISE 48

SHAKE IT OFF

In this exercise, you are going to shake each part of your body to release any tension or anxiety. This is perfect for when you have a lot of energy from the day that you need to release before bedtime.

1. Set a timer for 8 minutes.
2. Stand perfectly still with your feet parallel to each other. Relax your arms down by your sides.
3. Lift your right leg off the ground and shake it as you slowly count to 10.
4. Place your right foot back down on the ground.
5. Lift your left leg and shake it as you slowly count to 10.
6. Place your left foot back down on the ground.
7. Bring your attention to your left arm. Shake your arm as you slowly count to 10.
8. Bring your attention to your right arm. Shake your arm as you slowly count to 10.
9. Stand perfectly still and close your eyes. Count to 10 as you slowly inhale and exhale through your nose.

DID YOU KNOW?

When your body is stressed, it releases a hormone called cortisol. Cortisol produces anxiety and depression in your body. When you practice "shaking it off," you can reduce the amount of cortisol in your system.

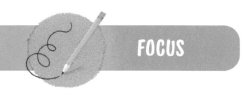

EXERCISE 49

STARRY NIGHT

The thoughts in our mind can twinkle like stars in the night sky. Some nights the sky can be filled with many stars, just as our minds can be filled with many thoughts. The more we focus on our thoughts, positive or negative, the bigger and brighter they will become. This meditation gives you the opportunity to use the stars as reminders to focus on your breathing. This exercise is best practiced outside at dusk, just as the sun has set and the sky is growing darker.

1. Find a spot outside to sit comfortably, then set a timer for 10 minutes.

2. Look up at the sky. Notice the colors as the sun is setting. How many colors do you see? Are they changing? Are they staying the same?

3. See if you notice any stars in the sky. Are they big or small? Are they getting brighter?

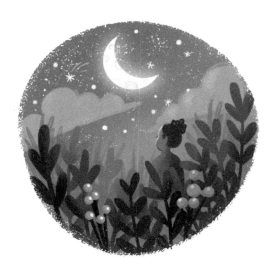

4. Pick one star. Focus your gaze on that star.

5. Inhale and exhale deeply through your nose as you focus on the star.

6. Look for another star. Inhale and exhale deeply through your nose.

7. Continue looking for new stars as you breathe deeply in and out through your nose.

WRITE AND REFLECT

Draw a picture of yourself, with the night sky above you. Try to remember the placement of the stars you focused on. Include the moon, if you could see it from where you were sitting. Did you notice any constellations? Put them in your drawing, too.

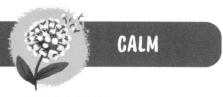

EXERCISE 50

SLEEPY BUTTERFLY

Did you know that monarch butterflies can travel up to 100 miles in one day? That's a lot of flying for those tiny wings. At the end of the day, they need to rest—just like you! This butterfly pose is great to practice before bedtime because it can help you feel calm and relaxed.

1. Set a timer for 5 minutes.
2. Sit on the floor. Bring the bottoms of your feet together so they touch in front of you.
3. Wrap your hands around your feet.
4. Sit up tall and inhale deeply through your nose.
5. Gently flap your legs up and down like the wings of a butterfly. Continue for three or four breaths, then let your legs relax into stillness.

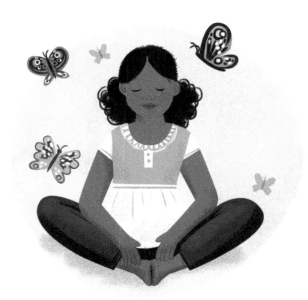

6. Exhale as you fold forward over your feet. Bring your nose toward your toes.

7. Count to 30 in your mind as you hold this position.

8. Inhale as you come back up to sit. Exhale as you fold over your feet again.

9. Repeat until the timer goes off.

GO DEEPER

While in your butterfly pose, you can use your hands to gently press down on your inner thighs. This will create a deeper stretch in your legs. First, take a slow, deep inhale. Then press gently on your thighs as you exhale. Do not push hard or force the stretch.

EXERCISE 51

FREEZE FRAME

Do you ever keep thinking about things that went wrong? Maybe it was something you said that you wish you hadn't. Maybe it was something you did that was embarrassing. Whatever it was, it *was*. That means it is in the past and you cannot change it. Instead of thinking of the situation in a negative way, you can look for something positive. This is called *reframing*. For example, if you said something you wish you hadn't, you can realize you've learned a lesson. You might have learned that you can choose your words more wisely in the future. If it was an embarrassing situation, maybe you gave your friends a good laugh. And maybe they really needed a good laugh that day! Whatever happened, we can reframe it.

1. Sit comfortably and set a timer for 5 minutes.
2. Breathe deeply in and out through your nose until you feel settled.
3. Think about an experience that made you feel bad or embarrassed. Picture it in your mind. Notice all the feelings it brings up in your body.
4. Reframe the experience with a positive thought. Repeat the thought to yourself as you breathe in and out through your nose. Allow any uncomfortable feelings in your body to melt away as you breathe.

5. If your mind goes back to a negative thought or situation, try again to reframe it with a positive thought.

6. Continue to breathe deeply in and out through your nose.

WRITE AND REFLECT

Things go wrong for people every day. It's a normal part of life! Make a list of things that went wrong for you today. Next to each item, reframe it by writing a positive thought or something you learned from that situation. Keep an ongoing list and reflect each week on how you reframed each situation. Reframing negative thoughts takes practice, but it will get easier over time.

EXERCISE 52

BEDTIME AFFIRMATIONS

How do you feel when someone notices your hard work or accomplishments? Like when your parents tell you they are proud of you, or when a teacher says, "Great job on your test!" It feels pretty good, right? Positive affirmations from others can make us feel good. But we can also feel good by saying positive things to ourselves. Practice this affirmation exercise as you settle into bed.

1. Lie down comfortably and set a timer for 8 minutes.

2. Breathe in and out through your nose.

3. Reflect on your day and think of something you love about yourself. For example, "I am brave," "I am smart," or "I am kind."

4. Repeat this positive affirmation in your mind.

DID YOU KNOW?

Practicing positive affirmations helps build confidence and self-esteem.

EXERCISE 53

TWIST IT OUT

At the end of a long day, you can relax your body for bedtime with a supine twist. *Supine* means lying on your back. When you do the twisting movements in this exercise with mindful breathing, you can release stress or tension that may have built up in your body during the day.

1. Set a timer for 8 minutes and lie on your back on the floor.

2. Bend your knees and place your feet flat on the floor.

3. Stretch your arms out wide like a giant letter T.

4. Bring your knees in toward your belly. Gently drop both knees over to the right side while keeping both shoulders flat on the floor.

5. Take a deep breath in and turn your head to the left.

6. Inhale and exhale three times.

7. On your next inhale, bring your knees back up to center. Gently drop them over to the left side while turning your head to the right.

8. Inhale and exhale three times.

> **GO DEEPER**
>
> Try the exercise with your eyes closed. Practicing a supine twist this way will help you focus more on your body and the sensations you are feeling with each twist. It may even help you get deeper into the twist and feel more relaxed.

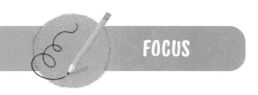

EXERCISE 54

COUNTDOWN TO SLEEP

Sometimes you cannot fall asleep at night, no matter how hard you try. There may be too many thoughts running through your head about what happened during the day, what will happen tomorrow, or all of it combined. You can focus your mind on something else by counting. This exercise can help settle your body for a great night's sleep.

1. Come to a comfortable sleep position. You may choose to set a timer for 8 minutes or practice with no timer.

2. As you breathe slowly in and out through your nose, feel your body settle into the bed.

3. Picture the number 10 in your mind as you inhale. Notice your body relax as you exhale.

4. Picture the number 9 in your mind as you inhale and exhale.

5. Continue counting down until you reach 0, inhaling and exhaling at each number.

6. If at any point your mind starts to wander and you lose count, simply begin again by starting at the number 10.

GO DEEPER

When practicing this countdown, you can set up your space for an even more relaxing experience. Dim the lights or turn them off completely and put on soft music in the background.

EXERCISE 55

YES, BUT

Have you ever had one of those days where it felt like everything went wrong? You woke up late, forgot to charge your computer the night before, there wasn't anything good to pack for lunch, you missed the bus, your best friend was out sick, and on and on. By the time you climb into bed at night you just feel defeated. Days like these are the best ones for this gratitude exercise. Practicing gratitude can help us see that even on our most challenging days, there is always something to be grateful for.

1. Sit comfortably and set a timer for 5 minutes.
2. Close your eyes. Breathe deeply in and out through your nose.
3. Think of something that happened today that was not so great. Maybe it was something that disappointed you.
4. Next, think of something about that disappointment that makes you grateful. For example, "I was disappointed I didn't have my favorite food for lunch, BUT I am grateful to my parents for taking the time to make me lunch."

5. Continue with any other experiences from the day.

6. When your timer goes off, take three deep breaths.

WRITE AND REFLECT

Create a "Yes, BUT" journal to keep track of all the things that you are grateful for. At the end of every day or week, or just when you feel like it, you can write about something that disappointed you, then list all the things you can think of that are positive about that thing. You might be surprised what you come up with! Writing in a gratitude journal will help relieve stress from your day and make you feel calm before bed.

CALM

EXERCISE 56

CHILD'S POSE

Child's pose is a resting position that helps us slow down and tune out distractions. It also helps to calm our minds and nervous systems, which makes it a great pose to practice before bedtime.

1. Set a timer for 5 minutes.

2. Come to kneel on the floor, then sit back on your heels.

3. Separate your knees wide, bringing your big toes to touch beneath you.

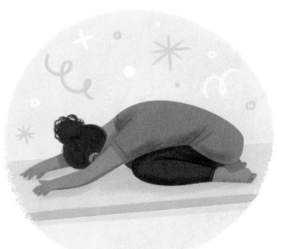

4. Fold forward and let your belly rest between your legs as you bring your forehead down to the floor.

5. Let your arms rest alongside your body.

6. Begin to breathe slowly in and out through your nose.

> **GO DEEPER**
>
> You can make your child's pose more active by reaching your arms forward instead of down by your sides.

EXERCISE 57

INHALE AND EXHALE

You can use your breath in different ways to either energize your body or calm it down. When you breathe in quickly, it energizes your body and makes your mind more alert. And when you exhale, it triggers the relaxation response in your brain that calms you. Have you ever noticed that after a big sigh your body feels relieved? That's your relaxation response kicking in. In this exercise, you will practice extending your exhales to relax the body and prepare for sleep.

1. Set a timer for 5 minutes.

2. Sit comfortably and close your eyes.

3. Slowly breathe in and out through your nose.

4. On your next inhale, count to two. On your exhale, count to four.

5. Continue breathing in this way, inhaling for two counts and exhaling for four counts.

6. If at any point your mind starts to wander, simply repeat your counting breaths.

7. When the timer goes off, resume your normal breathing pattern. Slowly open your eyes.

GO DEEPER

Practice extending each exhale. The next time you do this exercise, inhale for a count of three and exhale for a count of six. Always make the exhale count double the inhale count.

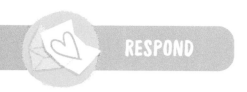

EXERCISE 58

PUT IT TO REST

Think about any worries you had today. Did worrying about those things help you? Did it make the worries go away? Probably not, right? You know worrying about things doesn't make them go away, and yet you just can't stop worrying. Or can you? By practicing mindfulness, you can learn to put those worries to rest at the end of each day, just like we put our bodies to rest in bed.

1. Sit comfortably and set a timer for 5 minutes.
2. Inhale and exhale through your nose.
3. Recall something that you worried about today.
4. Imagine tucking that worry away in a drawer. Once your worry is put away, take a deep breath in. Then exhale out through your nose.
5. Continue with any other worries you had throughout the day. One by one, put them all away in the drawer.
6. When you are finished, take a deep breath in through your nose and make an extended exhale out through your mouth with a sigh.

WRITE AND REFLECT

Keep a "worry journal" throughout the day. Every time a worry pops into your head, write it down. At the end of each day or week, review your worries and notice whether they are things you can change or not. Learning to let go of things outside of our control can help relieve some of those worries.

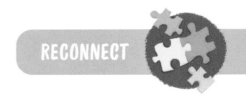
EXERCISE 59

HEART SHARING

A perfect way to end each day is with a heartfulness practice. In this exercise, you will send love and kind wishes to those you care about. By ending our day with kind thoughts for others, we are also filling ourselves with kindness. What a beautiful way to end your day!

1. Sit comfortably and set a timer for 8 minutes.
2. Place your hands, one on top of the other, over your heart.
3. Breathe slowly in and out through your nose.
4. Picture a person or people whom you love very much. See their faces in your mind.
5. On your next inhale, fill your heart with love for these people.
6. On your exhale, send all that love out to those people, wherever they may be.
7. Continue breathing in love and sending it out.
8. When you're finished, rest your hands on your lap and notice how you feel.

> **GO DEEPER**
> Repeat the exercise, but this time practice filling your heart with love for yourself.

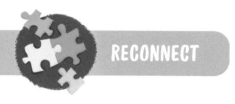
EXERCISE 60

BEDTIME MANTRA

At the end of a long day, do you think back to everything that happened or think about what you must do tomorrow? Try instead to focus on the present by reminding yourself that you have nowhere to be. This will help focus your mind on the present moment and calm your body for sleep.

1. Lie in a comfortable sleep position. You can set a timer for 5 minutes or practice this exercise without a timer.

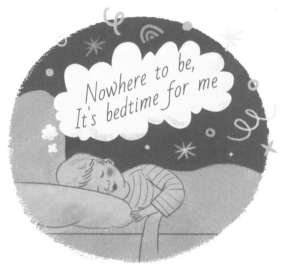

2. Close your eyes and breathe in and out through your nose.

3. Repeat the phrase "nowhere to be, it's bedtime for me" in your mind as you continue to breathe in and out through your nose.

4. With each exhale, imagine your body sinking deeper into your mattress. Feel it cradling you in warmth as you continue to repeat the phrase in your mind.

5. If at any point your mind starts to wander, simply bring it back by focusing on the words "nowhere to be, it's bedtime for me."

   GO DEEPER

   When you repeat a statement over and over in your mind, you are practicing a mantra. You can practice mantras any time you are feeling stressed. Try to come up with your own mantras to use throughout the day. You can try listing your positive traits (such as "I am brave" or "I am capable") or setting positive intentions (such as "This is going to be a great day" or "I'm going to have fun at the party").

"What day is it?" asked Pooh.
"It's today," squeaked Piglet.
"My favorite day," said Pooh.

—A. A. Milne

MINDFUL YOU

Go, You!

You did it! Congratulations for taking the time to work through the mindfulness exercises in this book. Whether you are brand-new to mindfulness or already practicing, you made a commitment to establishing positive habits. This will not only help you in the days ahead, but also in the weeks, months, and years, too!

By practicing the exercises in this book, you have learned mindfulness tools that can help you throughout each day. For instance, if you're stressed out about an upcoming test, you now know that mindful breathing can help you feel calm. If you had a fight with a friend and said something you regret, you can go back to one of the reconnect exercises to notice how you feel. Remember that by simply noticing how you feel, you are bringing your attention to the present moment, and that is mindfulness.

Think back to when you first opened this book. How were you feeling about mindfulness? What did you know about mindfulness? Now reflect on all you've read and practiced: breathing, walking, listening, seeing, eating.

How has it changed you? Has it changed you? Look back at any of your written reflections. Thank yourself for putting in this time and work. Notice how much you have grown in your mindfulness practice.

Don't Stop Now

You've come so far, so keep on going!

Now you have many mindfulness tools that are ready to use in an instant, whenever you need them. You have the power to calm yourself, to focus your mind, and to mindfully respond to any situation. You have the awareness of your body and how it feels. You are on your way to living more mindfully each day.

To improve or get better at anything, you must practice. By continuing to practice mindfulness, you will bring more calm, focus, gratitude, and happiness into your life. The mindfulness habit you have created will become second nature to you. Over time, you may find yourself naturally focusing on the present moment.

When things don't go your way or when bad things happen, you now have the tools to handle whatever comes your way. You can even create your own mindfulness exercises!

This is mindfulness.

MORE ON MINDFULNESS

BOOKS

Peaceful Piggy Meditation by Kerry Lee MacLean

A Pebble for Your Pocket: Mindful Stories for Children and Grown-ups by Thich Nhat Hanh

A Handful of Quiet: Happiness in Four Pebbles by Thich Nhat Hanh

Mindful Movements: Ten Exercises for Well-Being by Thich Nhat Hanh

I Am Peace: A Book of Mindfulness by Susan Verde

Listening to My Body by Gabi Garcia

Sitting Still Like a Frog: Mindfulness Exercises for Kids (and Their Parents) by Eline Snel

CARD DECKS

Card decks are so much fun to practice with! You just pick a single card and complete the exercise on the card. You can also pick a couple of cards to create your own yoga and mindfulness sequence.

Yoga and Mindfulness Practices for Children Card Deck by Jennifer Cohen Harper

The Mindful Yoga Breaks Card Deck by Lani Rosen-Gallagher and Jen Byer

APPS

Apps are a great way to continue your mindfulness practice. These apps include a variety of mindfulness activities plus timed meditations and sleep stories, which can help you focus and calm your mind and body.

Headspace
Smiling Mind
Stop, Breathe, Think
Insight Timer
Calm

Acknowledgments

I would like to thank all my teachers over the years who have shared their wisdom and gifts with me. Special thanks to YogaWorks, Little Flower Yoga, and Mindful Schools.

About the Author

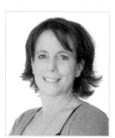 **Maura Bradley** is the owner and founder of Bee You Yoga, LLC, and formerly of Bee You kids yoga studio, which was in Manasquan, New Jersey. Maura is a certified adult and children's yoga teacher and a certified mindfulness instructor. Maura has been teaching kids yoga and mindfulness for more than 15 years and has taught thousands of children in weekly yoga and mindfulness classes, summer camps, schools, and specialty workshops. Currently, she is teaching kids yoga and mindfulness in schools throughout New Jersey and leads professional-development workshops for teachers, school staff, and administrators.

Maura currently lives on the Jersey Shore with her husband, Derek, their three kids, Emma, Will, and Maeve, and their dog, Jake.

CPSIA information can be obtained
at www.ICGtesting.com
Printed in the USA
BVHW051311050622
637827BV00004B/5